Cancer 101
THE TIME MACHINE
When Survival Seems Impossible

A H FITZSIMONS

Copyright © 2024 by A H FitzSimons

The right of A H FitzSimons to be identified as the author of this work has been asserted by him in accordance with the Copyright, Designs and Patents Act 1988

All rights reserved. No part of this publication may be reproduced, stored in a retrieval system, or transmitted in any other form or by any means, electronic, mechanical, photocopying, recording or otherwise without the prior written permission of the copyright holder

Published by Open Path Books 2024 ISBN 978-1-8383829-5-7
openpathbooks1@aol.com

Cover: OZZY EYRE

Acknowledgements

I thank Major (Retd) Ian Johnson, Rubén Manso, George Boyle, Ozzy Eyre and Ronald Hough for their assistance and encouragement during the writing of this short book.

Contents

Author's Note	7
Overview	9
The Strategy: Primary Assault	14
Second Assault	17
Obstacles: Pain and Lack of Self-belief	18
The Mind when both Assaults are Working Together	23
Sources	29
About the Author	31

Author's Note

I feel it is important to stress that although my recovery was deemed impossible it was not due to one factor but a combination of many, in particular the outstanding medical and nursing care I received during my stays in the Western General Hospital in Edinburgh: Dr Martin Eastwood being in charge of my care in 1994, and Mr D C C Bartolo (supported by Dr Mike Mackie) in 2003/4.

Overview

In 1994, following an acute flare up of ulcerative colitis the author survived a two-month spell in hospital against all medical expectation. He became unwell again in the fall of 2000. Certain it was colitis he continued on appropriate medication until being admitted to hospital in February 2003 which led to an operation to remove his large intestine. During the operation he was found to be suffering not from colitis but advanced non-Hodgkin's lymphoma, the disease having been active for more than two years. In the months that followed he underwent a further four major operations including an emergency operation to remove a kidney, suffered a number of complications including a blood clot on the lung, and a brain stem stroke when a 'do not resuscitate' order was placed on him. Shortly after this, treatment for the lymphoma was found to be totally ineffective. It was at this point, at less than half his normal bodyweight, the doctors deemed survival impossible.

This short book details the same mental strategy the author employed during both stays in hospital, a strategy that was complementary to the professional treatment he received. Although this strategy was right for him, he is reluctant to recommend it to anyone else. When asked he makes reference to the film *Zero Dark Thirty*. Based on actual events the film shows 'enhanced interrogation techniques' being used to extract information from a terrorist. Enhanced interrogation techniques were developed after the 9/11 terrorist attacks. These techniques were clearly methods of torture, where prisoners were made to feel fear and extremes of pain and discomfort. The prisoners would eventually learn they had no control over anything and would lose belief in themselves. Unable to offer any mental or physical resistance, they would accept the role of victim.

The author saw that all too often it is the same process with serious illness. In homes and hospitals all over the world patients have their confidence broken by fear, sleep deprivation and prolonged and extreme pain and discomfort. Without direction they learn how helpless they are. When a patient accepts the role of victim, the body's immune system is often suppressed, healing mechanisms can shut down and the illness, fuelled by the nocebo effect (the opposite of the placebo effect), can take over.

There is, however, an important difference between the two scenarios – those who are taken prisoner are often well prepared for the torture. The so-called 'enhanced techniques' were devised by reverse-engineering the SERE programme (Survival, Evasion, Resistance and Escape) taught to US military who were at risk of being captured by the enemy. Funding is huge: the budget set for reverse-engineering the SERE programme was over US $180 million. The UK military runs its own equivalent to SERE. Yet when so much money is invested in training the military, for an event they will probably never encounter, there is a near total lack of education and preparation for the countless patients who, after diagnosis, suddenly find themselves in the middle of a psychological war zone. This is hardly surprising, though, when you consider the sheer mass of information that is available on how to combat cancer. Moreover, the problem is not solely that there is too much information, but also that too much of it is contradictory.

The author felt that a short, straightforward guidebook could be helpful. Despite his reluctance to recommend such an extreme strategy he does feel that understanding aspects of it could be beneficial for patients to assist in developing their own strategy, one that is right for them as individuals.

Relevant Research Findings:

Being on long term immune system suppressants is recognized as being one of the causes for developing cancer, as are prolonged periods of trauma/stress. It is a clear indication of the importance of the immune system – a lowering of immune function can result in the development of cancer yet the opposite is also true – increasing immune function will help in combating cancer.

A typical reaction to a diagnosis of cancer or life-threatening illness is an immediate loss of control, and the negative thoughts and emotions that accompany it: fear, depression and despair.

Anger can suppress immune function for hours. Fear, depression and despair also suppress immune function.

From the vast amount of research on the placebo effect we know that believing in recovery (regardless of how that belief is attained) will reduce/negate destructive emotions like fear and depression, and will boost immune function and trigger healing mechanisms.

Feelings of love and compassion boost immune function within minutes.

Research suggests that mirthful laughter not only boosts immune function but can increase the production of killer cells (cells that target and kill cancer cells).

Total belief, total faith in an outcome is a common denominator in cases of spontaneous healing, commonly known as miracles.

We can say with confidence that striving to attain the highest level of belief in recovery, taking as much enjoyment out of life as possible, being around people we love and those who make us laugh would, when combined with expert medical care, be the perfect way to combat illness and give us the best chance of a fast recovery.

However, if our prognosis is unfavourable we will be wary of believing, we will look for proof as to whether such a strategy will work with cancer. And of course, the kind of proof we're looking for, the hard evidence, is still limited. But the lack of evidence is irrelevant because there isn't any proof, any hard evidence to say it won't work, as long it is combined with expert medical care.

Research isn't about certainty – it is about direction. It gives us a path to follow, a path that if we persevere with, will reduce and potentially negate destructive thoughts, boost the immune system and enhance medication. A path that allows us to reach out for a seemingly impossible goal – spontaneous healing, a miracle, via total belief, acceptance, that recovery is a certainty. Even if we don't reach that level of acceptance, we will reap the benefits from the belief we attain on the journey.

So we have a path to follow, but how do we believe, especially when our bodies are betraying us and our self-belief is at an all time low? Due to the close relationship between self-belief and the ability to believe, to simply believe in a desired future is a hard ask. Where do we start? How can we begin to regain control?

The Strategy

First objective/primary assault:

Regain a level of control by establishing a routine based around the work of psychologist Jean Achterberg.

Professor Achterberg could determine with 93 per cent precision which of her patients would recover and which would get worse and die purely from rating their visualizations. The recovery group were those who had a greater ability to visualize vividly, convincingly and regularly.

Visualization is a way of redirecting the mind. Redirection is an art frequently used by magicians – more commonly, albeit incorrectly, known as 'misdirection' – what the eyes see, and the ears hear, the mind believes.

The 'redirection' occurs because the brain's visual cortex (the area responsible for processing images) cannot tell the difference between what is vividly imagined and what is real.

Yet we have a problem with visualization. When we are unwell, visualizing ourselves as healthy in the future seems impossible. However, the one thing we can do is flash an image from the future. That is possible, even if it is only for a fraction of a second.

What would that image be?

What is the future we would most want to have, to live? Imagine that future for a second then create a snapshot, an image or images that encapsulate it. The choice is important as this snapshot, or snapshots, will be flashed in the mind as often as possible. Ideally, we will be able to a develop this image into a short film of a few seconds but for now a snapshot that represents our desired future will be used.

An example of image/film: seeing the confidence in your consultant's expression when he gives you the all clear and the unbridled joy in your partner's face.

There is research which indicates that visualization should be gradual, and the focus should be on one stage at a time. This could take the form of looking at the first in a series of scan or blood results. However, the strategy detailed in this book would miss those visualizations out completely – the focus and emphasis being on the end result. An athlete may visualize winning each of the next 20 races he has to compete in to get to the Olympics in four years' time. But if he employed this strategy he would miss those races out, instead focusing on the actual Olympics and repeatedly visualizing himself standing on the podium with the gold medal around his neck. When he was able to develop this into a film he would see his country's flag being raised, hear himself singing the national anthem, feel the cool breeze against his face accompanied by an acute sense of national pride.

Images and films played out in the mind form the primary assault to redirect the mind to believe in a desired future as opposed to a future dictated by illness.

We want to believe because of the benefits of believing, but belief will take time. However, there are immediate benefits to engaging in this the first assault: the mind now has a goal, a purpose, and is active. Engaging our minds in a positive manner keeps our thoughts from wandering and allowing symptoms of the illness to lead us to destructive thoughts.

By staying busy, by actively working, we are starting the process of restoring self-belief which has been decimated by diagnosis and the knowledge that our bodies are betraying us. We are also, importantly, starting to regain a level of control.

Second assault:

This is in addition to the primary assault. In effect it is the equivalent of opening up the attack on cancer on an additional front. We continue to flash images of our desired future, which can be one image, or now, several images, or short films. In doing so we are reinforcing what is becoming an established routine. The second assault takes a less direct route, via deception: the goal being to trick the mind into accepting we have already recovered by thinking and acting (as far as possible) that we have done precisely that.

An example of this may be starting to plan what we will do when we get the all clear. For example: go on a deep-sea fishing trip, except instead of waiting until we get the all clear, pretend we already have it. So we commence organizing the trip, looking through brochures, surfing the net, checking out, and identifying the best company to go with. Speaking to the friends who will accompany us on the trip. Going into detail, what equipment we will need, what clothing, which hotel/s we will stay in. Once that's all planned, the images and films of these plans unfolding in the future, i.e. on the trip itself, automatically become part of our film library used in the primary assault.

Obstacles: Pain and Lack of Self-Belief

Pain

At a TEDx talk in Adelaide, neuroscientist Lorimer Moseley spoke about the processes of pain and the reasons 'why things hurt'. Moseley described two experiences with pain. The first was felt when walking with friends through the Australian bush and something grazed against his bare leg. He described how this activated receptors on the end of fast-conducting nerve fibres which went straight up his leg into the spinal cord, and from there up to the brain giving notification that something had touched the skin on his leg. Meanwhile, at the actual site on the leg, the activity was sufficiently intense to activate free nerve endings which sent a message to the spinal cord that something dangerous had happened to the leg at the point where contact was made. This then passed a message to the spinal cord which relayed to the brain a warning of danger. The brain now had to assess the level of danger and determine if action must be taken. Different areas of the brain, performing different tasks, assessed the neural information.

In this case, no fight or flight triggers were activated by the neural processing: Moseley had been in the same environment before on many occasions and had experienced a similar event with no dangerous outcome. On this occasion, the warning signals were dismissed and the pain faded into insignificance.

Moseley had, in fact, been bitten by a highly poisonous snake and not, as he assumed, scratched by a twig; he collapsed soon afterwards.

The second experience was six months later when Moseley was walking through the bush again. This time a similar thing happened; the same processes were activated from the site of contact to the spinal cord and to the brain. However, when the brain assessed the danger by asking if he had been in this environment before, as opposed to remembering an earlier experience of being grazed by a twig, the brain determined that this was probably a snake bite and sent extreme warning signals that this was serious – the pain, this time, was horrendous. Moseley felt agonising pain until one of his friends examined his leg and announced that he had merely been scratched by a twig.

The pain Moseley felt was a direct reflection of his perception of the danger.

Cancer, as with several other life-threatening illnesses, typically leads to patients suffering considerable pain. This alone leads to destructive thoughts, made worse when pain prevents us from sleeping. However, we possess the potential to exert control over the assessment process for different levels of pain. We have a say in our interpretation of, and meaning we give to, the warning signals; and the level and duration of these signals, in other words, the pain itself. If we can switch off the warning signals, for example by accepting that the pain is necessary for survival, we take a level of control over the pain. This level of control will be heightened if we can program our desired future when we're in pain, and doing so will automatically build self-belief.

It is possible to take something beneficial from pain. Using pain by ignoring the warning signals whilst under medical supervision carries little danger. However, adopting this approach without anyone to watch over us, carries the risk of doing something extremely dangerous. If we make an error in diagnosis, it could prove fatal.

Self-belief

There has been a growing trend in Sports Psychology concerning the importance of self-belief. Hardly surprising, as there is a consensus that the more confident the sportsman or woman, the better they perform. In 2001 a research study was conducted into what factors helped ten of the world's top athletes excel in their sport: at the top of the list were unshakable self-belief in their own ability and the conviction they possessed qualities that made them better than their opponents.

A 2014 BBC episode of *Horizon* entitled, 'The Power of the Placebo', gives insight into this subject. The programme attempted to establish whether the placebo effect was imagined, or if actual changes were taking place in the body. An experiment was conducted at high altitude where, in the middle of a trek, the test subject was led to believe he was being given oxygen but was, in fact, being given placebo oxygen, in other words, normal air.

At high altitude the low oxygen level in the air causes a lowering of the oxygen level in the blood; this, in turn, brings about an increase in the level of the neurotransmitter PGE2, which results in pain. When the test subject received the placebo oxygen, oxygen levels in his blood remained the same. However, there was a lowering of PGE2, allowing an increase in physical performance as his pain levels dropped.

This was not an imagined response. The fake oxygen didn't give a psychological boost, real physiological changes took place.

The *Horizon* episode, 'The Power of the Placebo', could equally have been called, 'The Power of Belief'. The placebo is something tangible that generates belief: the starch or sugar tablet or the fake oxygen are stepping stones to belief in a certain outcome which results in physical change. Self-belief can do the same without the stepping stones. It is accepted that self-belief is necessary for athletes and sportsmen/women to give them the confidence to beat their opponents. Yet, it is not widely accepted that self-belief brings about chemical changes which allow the body to perform at a higher level. This is partly because the line between a psychological boost and physiological change is difficult to identify. A second wind is still regarded as just that, something intangible; but, in the military, many know what is involved.

Soldiers in Special Forces units have colossal egos: combat orientated, they live for their profession and that means being able to push themselves harder than anyone else. These soldiers exhibit what is commonly known as 'Superman Syndrome'. If you put one of them through an endurance test at high altitude, PGE2 levels would most likely fall, but without placebo oxygen being administered. It would simply be a case of moving to another level of endurance. The first day of selection for Special Forces candidates eliminates all those who don't have the ability to break through their pain barriers.

The strongman Joe Greenstein, who at 83 performed feats of strength to three standing ovations at Madison Square Garden, knew the importance of self-belief. Before attempting to bend a thick iron bar, he would hold the bar in his hands and accept that he was stronger than it.

Herschel Walker, the near unstoppable running back, did not only see himself as faster and stronger than anyone else, he saw himself as superhuman: as someone who was capable of anything when he had the ball.

There are numerous examples of those who accomplish feats that appear impossible, Greenstein being perhaps the most extreme example, standing five feet four inches and weighing around 140 pounds he refused to put limits on himself. He featured frequently in the Guinness Book of Records, and also the Press for his fights against those who abuse power where he was always outnumbered, yet always the one left standing.

We all have the potential to access a legal performance-enhancing drug – we just need the confidence in ourselves to take it.

Self-belief and self-esteem are essential for believing in a desired future. We may be able to imagine the future of our dreams, but we won't truly believe in that future without a strong sense of self-belief and self-worth that allows us to feel we are worthy of that future.

The Mind when both Assaults are Working Together

We know the human brain functions like a sophisticated computer. It therefore follows that in order to re-direct it to accept a desired future, we have to re-program it.

It actually helps, considering our physical condition and what we are trying to achieve, to think of ourselves as machines. When we wake, or surface from the drugs, when the machine is switched on, it runs its start-up program: identifying its purpose, its primary directive. Then the machine searches through its memory banks, ignoring anything that conflicts with this directive until it finds the data that support it, forcing itself into playing its main program – images of the future – until it uses up its power supply, at which point it shuts down. Some time later (whether that is minutes, hours or days) the machine is switched on again.

It is an ideal. Even without the pain and discomfort, it is an impossible ideal. Yet it is a goal; it gives us something to aim at.

By reprogramming and redirecting the mind, we can, in time, create a future reality; yet we're still in the present. We've been functioning effectively as a time machine, delving in to the future every day and in doing so we are now existing between two opposing, conflicting, realities.

Our mind struggles to cope with these two realities. It will want to accept one, reject the other, and put an end to the war. It's far easier to accept the reality that we've been conditioned to accept from childhood. Our mind will naturally attempt to accept the present and the fearful future that seems destined to unfold from it. In direct conflict to that is the reality of the strategy which says if we persevere with programming our desired future and pretending that future is a certainty, we will survive. The conflict is heightened with logic asking, 'but where is the proof that we will survive?' Against that, the logic of the strategy will respond: 'we committed ourselves to this path aware there was no definite proof. We accepted that it was going to be difficult; we must find a way to persevere.'

If we allow it to, the argument will rage on every day as our mind attempts to find an answer that makes sense. Those days will be wasted with no programming and no pretending, eventually leading to the strategy breaking down. The only answer is a determined refusal to engage in argument by ignoring the inner voice that demands we do, and thus persevering with our strict routine. By relentlessly programming our desired future, we are striving to force our mind into accepting that future. If we achieve this, then the mind has to accept recovery.

That's both the key and vulnerability of this strategy. We need to persevere, but the way we redirect the mind via a combination of two assaults means the programming must be relentless. If we're not programming, then we should at least be striving to think as though we've already recovered, or that recovery is a certainty. In this sense it's all about momentum. If we're not looking forward to the future, then present reality could begin to dominate. As a result, we may lose momentum and with it the level of belief we've worked hard to attain.

Relentless programming and persevering require a level of commitment, and the start point of the strategy is to understand the true level that's necessary. We cannot be at the mercy of feedback, because recovery is not a straight line going upwards. It is a seesaw of ups and downs, and at various stages we're going to be hit hard not just by a lack of positive feedback but by negative feedback. If we can place the act of persevering as more important than survival, then feedback, positive or negative, will become irrelevant.

The level of self-discipline required for this strategy is extreme. Perseverance in the sense of enduring is not enough, we're talking about substituting one reality (the present) for another (the future). That in itself is going to be difficult, even more so when the present will possibly be bombarding us with reminders of its existence in the form of pain and discomfort.

To stay on course, to refuse to question or doubt takes an incredibly high level of confidence, not just in the strategy, but in ourselves. Although the strategy builds self-belief via hard work, it may not be enough – we should use anything we can to build self-belief.

For example, we feel we have failed ourselves, or others, by making mistakes, or by not fighting when really we should have. If we do have regrets, if we have guilt, we now finally have a chance of redemption. Redemption achieved by fighting now. In fighting to persevere no matter what, in pushing ourselves harder than we ever thought possible, we fight the fights we failed to fight in the past.

We can also build self-belief by recalling past achievements, moments where we have been proud of our actions. If we don't have them, then we take them from the future, from the vows made of what we're going to achieve. Picturing these achievements in our mind will give us images and films we can add to the library of footage we use in the primary assault.

The strategy, initially occupying the mind to stop it wandering to destructive thoughts, builds belief in ourselves and in a fast recovery, whilst constantly reaching out for acceptance that our desired future is a certainty. In theory it will be fuelled by adversity. The more obstacles illness throws at us the more we have to program, and in doing so, we naturally build self-belief. Via total commitment there is no alternative path, and in this lies the danger inherent in the strategy. In building belief in our desired future we also build a cauldron of despair. If we stop, we suffer the loss of belief, and all the horrors that might entail. The stronger the belief, potentially the greater the despair. We may use that knowledge as a way of forcing ourselves to continue, but if we fail to persevere we may fall into the cauldron.

Before committing to a strategy of this nature we must be aware of, and accept, the risk that goes with it.

To quote Norman Mailer: 'Great hope has no real footing unless one is willing to face into the doom that may also be on the way.'

If we are willing to accept the risk involved and manage to persevere with programming, and pretending our desired future is a certainty; if we can see through the long days where there is no positive feedback, and the even longer days of negative feedback; if we can use the pain, to help build our self-belief to the point that we become indifferent to things going wrong we may, in time, find ourselves daydreaming of our desired future; then we have reached the point where we're starting to truly believe and our desired future is dominating. Up until this point the strategy has been hard work. Now we can take pleasure from the feeling of euphoria that accompanies our daydreams. There are no guarantees with any strategy, but we have, through all the days and nights of mental combat, reached the point where we are at one with ourselves – we have done what we set out to do. Survival would, in theory, be a by-product of expert medical care in combination with the strategy (although the extent of the role played by the strategy would never be known). Then we would be duty-bound to fulfil the promises and vows we made. From experience there's no escaping them. You're reading my vow; it just took me twenty years to finish writing it.

Sources

Achterberg, J., & Lawlis, G.F. (1980). *Bridges of the Bodymind: Behavioural Approaches for Health Care*, Champaign, IL: Institute for Personality and Ability Testing.

Alternative Medicine: The Evidence (2006) [Television documentary]. BBC2, 24 January, 21:00.

Bennett, M.P., Zeller, J.M., Rosenberg, L., & McCann, J. (2003). The Effect of Mirthful Laughter on Stress and Natural Killer Cell Activity. *Alternative Therapies in Health and Medicine, 9*(2), 38-45.

Brody, H. (2000). *The Placebo Response.* New York: HarperCollins.

Cooper, W., & Smith, T. (1981). *Human Potential: The Limits and Beyond*, Newton Abbot, David and Charles Publishers.

Cornwell, J. (2000, December 24). Trick or treatment? *The Sunday Times Magazine,* 23-28.

Cornwell, J. (2009, September 23). The drugs don't work. *Prospect.* Retrieved from Prospect magazine http://www.prospectmagazine.co.uk/features/the-drugs-don't-work-2

Horizon (2014) [Television series episode]. The Power of the Placebo. BBC2, February 13, 21:00.

Ikemi, Y., & Nakagawa, S. (1962). Skin reactivity with hypnotic induction: A psychosomatic study of contagious dermatitis. *Kyushu Journal of Medical Science, 13,* 335-350

Jones, G. (2002). What Is This Thing Called Mental Toughness? An Investigation of Elite Sport Performers. *Journal of Applied Sports Psychology, 14*(3), 205-218.

Moseley, L. (2011, November 22). Why things hurt [Video file]. Retrieved from:
    https://www.youtube.com/watch?v=gwd-wLdIHjs.

Rein, G., Atkinson, M., & McCraty, R. (1995). The physiological and psychological effects of compassion and anger. *Journal of Advancement in Medicine, 8,* 87-105.

Spielman, E. (1979). *The Mighty Atom: The Life and Times of Joseph L. Greenstein.* New York: Viking Press.

Touching the Void (2003) [Film]. Kevin McDonald (Director). United Kingdom: Film Four.

About the author

Anton Hugh FitzSimons (pen name A H FitzSimons) was born in Johnstone, near Glasgow, in 1958. He served in the British Army in the 1970s and 1980s before joining Lothian and Borders Police. He studied at Telford and Napier Colleges in Edinburgh, winning two Scottish Business Education Council Awards, including the C.A. Oakley gold medal, before graduating in 1988. Following his sixteen-month stay in hospital he wrote the non-fictional book *The Fight* (2007), detailing the mental conflict he underwent in employing the strategy on a day-to-day basis. However, he felt he had failed to fully explain the strategy and attempted to rectify this with *Extreme Mental Combat* (2016) and *Total War: Maximizing the Body's Own Resources* (2020). [He deemed both books as additional failures and withdrew them from distribution.] He also tried to incorporate aspects of the strategy into several fictional books namely *The Game* (2012), *Break Lima* (2014) and *HK9* (2022) eventually breaking away from the subject altogether with *Not Proven: Fair Game* (2023). In 2024 he returned to the strategy again. In addition to this short guidebook, he updated his first book publishing it as *The Fight: 2024* whilst leaving the original 2007 version available in print and eBook.

www.ingramcontent.com/pod-product-compliance
Lightning Source LLC
Chambersburg PA
CBHW050156130526
44590CB00044B/3369